Veggie Soups and Salads

A Quick and Easy Cooking Guide for Your Vegetarian Daily Meals

Kaylee Collins

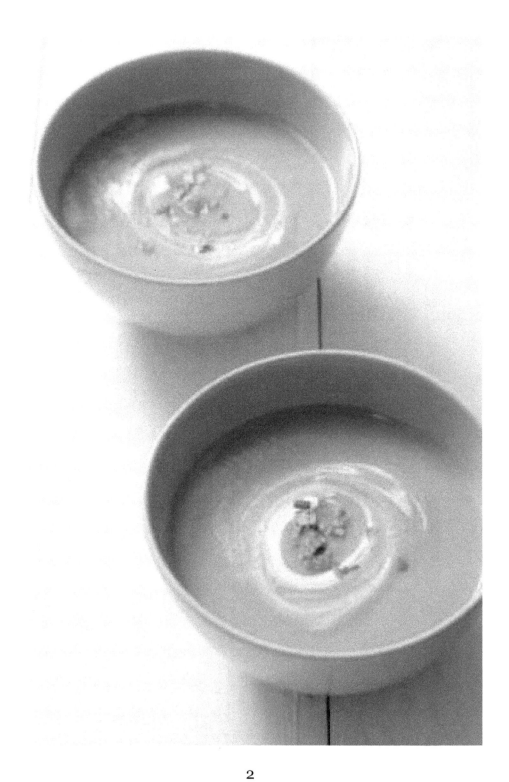

Table of Contents

Easy Keto Tomato Basil Soup 6

Low Carb Cream of Broccoli & Cheddar Soup 9

Ginger zucchini noodle egg drop soup 11

Anti-Inflammatory Egg Drop Soup 13

Soy Bean and Bell Pepper Soup 15

Mexican Spaghettini Soup 17

Split Pea Celery and Leek Soup 19

Red Potato and Baby Spinach Soup 20

Garnish with lemon Slow Cooked Lima Bean Soup 21

Carrot and Cardamom Soup 23

Borlotti Bean Soup 26

Lentil Soup 28

Triple Bean Soup 30

Parsnips and Summer Squash Soup 32

Butternut Squash and Apple Soup 34

Summer Squash and Apple Soup 36

Chinese Butternut Squash Soup 38

Pinto Beans and Olives Tortilla Soup 40

Butterbean Taco Soup 42

Jalapeno and Soybean Taco Soup 44

Navy Bean and Jalapeno Pepper Soup 46

Pigeon Peas Soup 48

Chia Seeds Tomato Soup 50

Zucchini Soup 52

Anise Seed and Cabbage Soup 54

Bok Choy Soup 56

Spicy Peanut Soup with Potato and Spinach 58

Parsnip Ginger Soup with Tofu and Kale 60

Mushroom Soup 63

Seitan Stew with Barley 65

Cottage Cheese Soup 67

Cauliflower Soup 69

Pumpkin Soup 71

Vegetarian Spinach Soup 73

Green Soup 75

Zoodles Greek Salad 77

Antipasto Cauliflower Salad 79

Charred Veggie and Fried Goat Cheese Salad 81

Simple Greek Salad 83

Keto Asian Noodle Salad with Peanut Sauce 85

Crispy Tofu and Bok Choy Salad 88

Low-Carb Snap Pea Salad 91

Black Bean Salad with Apricots 94

Red Potato Salad 96

Awesome Pasta Salad 98

Brown Lentil Salad with dill 100

Cucumber, Mango, and Barley Salad 102

Greek Green Bean Salad with Feta and Tomatoes 104

Quick Edamame Salad 106

Green Bean and Potato Salad 108

Easy Keto Tomato Basil Soup

A creamy and delicious low carb tomato soup recipe that takes just minutes to prepare! Keto, Atkins, and gluten free – this is an easy and tasty soup that you can feel great about serving to your family!

Prep Time: 2 minutes Cook Time: 10 minutes Total Time: 12 minutes Servings: 6 servings

Ingredients

1 can (28 ounces) whole plum tomatoes (San Marzano preferred)

2 cups filtered water

1.5 teaspoons coarse kosher salt

1/2 teaspoon onion powder

1/4 teaspoon garlic powder

1 tablespoon butter

8 ounces mascarpone cheese

2 tablespoons granulated erythritol sweetener

1 teaspoon apple cider vinegar

1/4 teaspoon dried basil leaves

1/4 cup prepared basil pesto, plus more for garnish if desired

Instructions

Combine the canned tomatoes, water, salt, onion powder and garlic powder in a medium saucepan.

Bring to a boil over medium-high heat and then simmer for 2 minutes.

Remove from the heat and puree with an immersion blender until smooth (or transfer to a traditional blender and blend, then return blended soup to the pan.)

Return to the stove and add the butter and mascarpone cheese to the soup.

Stir over low heat until melted and creamy – about 2 minutes. Remove from the heat and stir in the sweetener, apple cider vinegar, dried basil, and pesto.

Serve warm.

Store any leftovers in a covered container in the refrigerator for up to 5 days, or in the freezer for up to three months.

Nutrition Info

Serving Size: 1 cup Calories: 258

Fat: 23g Carbohydrates: 6g Fiber: 3g

Protein: 4g

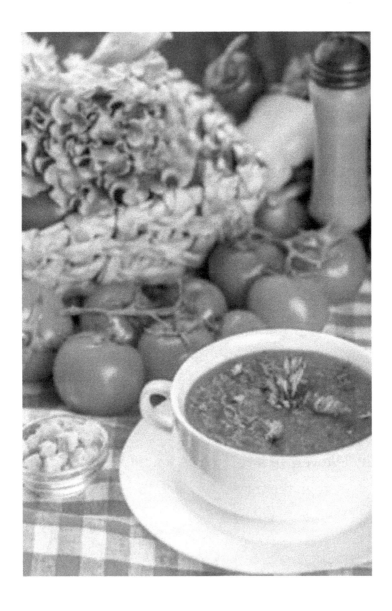

Low Carb Cream of Broccoli & Cheddar Soup

Ingredients

4 cups broccoli florets

2 cups beef broth

1 cup sharp cheddar cheese, shredded

1/2 tsp garlic powder

 1/2 tsp onion powder

1/2 tsp mustard powder

1/8 tsp nutmeg

1/2 tsp kosher salt (or to taste)

1/4 tsp ground black pepper

1/2 cup heavy whipping cream

1/4 cup butter

Instructions

Cook the broccoli florets for 4 minutes in the microwave on high (or steam them on the stove.) Combine the broccoli and other ingredients in a blender and blend until mostly smooth.

Cook on high in the microwave for 2 minutes, stir and cook another 2 minutes, repeat one more time and serve hot.

Alternatively, simmer in a pot on the stove for about 10 minutes. Serve hot.

Nutrition Info

255 calories 22g fat

3g net carbs 7g protein

Ginger zucchini noodle egg drop soup

Prep Time: 10 minutes Cook Time: 15 minutes Total Time: 25 minutes Servings: 4-6 servings

Ingredients

4 medium to large zucchini

2 tablespoons extra virgin olive oil 2 tablespoons minced ginger

5 cups shiitake mushrooms, sliced 8 cups vegetable broth, divided

2 cups, plus 1 tablespoon water, divided 1/2 teaspoons red pepper flakes

5 tablespoons low-sodium tamari sauce or soy sauce 2 cups thinly sliced scallions, divided

4 large eggs, beaten

1 tablespoons corn starch Salt & pepper to taste

Instructions

Prepare the zucchini noodles with a spiralizer using the step- by-step guide above.

In a large pot, heat the olive oil over medium-high heat. Add the minced ginger and cook, stirring, for 2 minutes.

Add the shiitake mushrooms and a tablespoon of water and cook until the mushrooms begin to sweat.

Add 7 cups of the vegetable broth, the remaining water, the red pepper flakes, tamari sauce, and 1½ cups of the chopped scallions. Bring to a boil, stirring occasionally.

Meanwhile, mix the remaining cup of vegetable broth with the corn starch and whisk until completely smooth.

While stirring the soup, slowly pour in the beaten eggs in a thin stream. Continue stirring until all of the egg is incorporated.

Slowly pour the corn starch mixture into the soup and cook for about 4-5 minutes to thicken.

Season to taste with salt & pepper (usually I add just a bit of pepper, but as long, as I'm using a full-sodium vegetable broth, I don't need any extra salt).

Add the spiralized zucchini noodles to the pot and cook, stirring, for about 2 minutes, or until the noodles are just soft and flexible (remember, they'll continue cooking in your bowl!).

Serve topped with the remaining scallions.

Anti-Inflammatory Egg Drop Soup

Hands-on 10 minutes Total Time: 20 minutes Serving 2 cups/ 480 ml

Ingredients (makes 6 servings)

2 quarts (2 l) chicken stock or vegetable stock or bone broth - you can make your own

1 tbsp freshly grated turmeric or 1 tsp ground turmeric 1 tbsp freshly grated ginger or 1 tsp ground ginger

2 cloves garlic, minced

1 small chile pepper, sliced (14 g/ 0.5 oz) 2 tbsp coconut aminos

2 cups sliced brown mushrooms (144 g/ 5.1 oz)

4 cups chopped Swiss chard or spinach (144 g/ 5.1 oz) 4 large eggs

2 medium spring onions, sliced (30 g/ 1.1 oz) 2 tbsp freshly chopped cilantro

1 tsp salt or to taste (I like pink Himalayan) freshly ground black pepper to taste

6 tbsp extra virgin olive oil (90 ml/ 3 fl oz)

Instructions

Grate the turmeric and ginger root, slice the chile pepper and mince the garlic cloves. Anti-Inflammatory Egg Drop Soup Pour the chicken stock (or vegetable stock) in a large pot and heat over a medium heat, until it starts to simmer. Slice the mushrooms, ... Anti-Inflammatory Egg Drop Soup

... chard stalks and chard leaves. Place the turmeric, ginger, garlic, chile pepper, mushrooms, chard stalks and coconut aminos into the pot and simmer for about 5 minutes. Anti-Inflammatory Egg Drop Soup.

Then add the sliced chard leaves and cook for another minute. In a bowl, whisk the eggs and slowly pour them into the simmering soup. Anti-Inflammatory Egg Drop Soup.

Keep stirring until the egg is cooked and take off the heat. Chop the cilantro and slice the spring onions. Add them to the pot. Season with salt and pepper to taste. Anti-Inflammatory Egg Drop Soup.

Pour into a serving bowl and drizzle with extra virgin olive oil (a tablespoon per serving). Eat immediately or let it cool down and store in an airtight container for up to 5 days.

Soy Bean and Bell Pepper Soup

Ingredients

1 pound dry soy beans

4 cups vegetable stock

1 yellow onion, finely chopped

1 green bell pepper, finely chopped

2 jalapeños, seeds removed and finely chopped

1 cup salsa or diced tomatoes

4 teaspoons minced garlic, about 4 cloves

1 heaping tablespoon chili powder

2 teaspoons ground cumin

2 teaspoons sea salt

1 teaspoon ground pepper

1/2 teaspoon ground cayenne pepper (decrease or omit for a milder soup)

1/2 teaspoon smoked paprika

Avocado and cilantro for topping, if desired

Directions:

Completely submerge the beans in water overnight and make sure there's an inch of water over the beans. Drain the beans and rinse. Put the beans, broth, onion, pepper, jalapeños, salsa, garlic, chili powder, cumin, salt, pepper, cayenne, and paprika in a slow cooker. Stir and combine thoroughly. Cook on high heat for 6 hours until beans are tender. Blend half of the soup until smooth and bring it back to the pot. Top with avocado and cilantro.

Mexican Spaghettini Soup

Ingredients

5 large tomatoes, cut into large cubes

1 medium red onion, cut into large cubes

3 cloves garlic

2 Tbsp. olive oil

16 oz. spaghettini, broken into 1-inch pieces

32 oz. vegetable broth

1/2 tsp. sea salt

1/2 Tbsp. black pepper

2 Tbsp. oregano

2 Tbsp. cumin Chili flakes, chopped Serrano chilies, or diced jalapeños, to taste (optional)

Directions:

Cilantro, sour soy cream, and sliced avocado for garnish (optional) Puree the tomatoes, red onions, garlic, and oil. Transfer to a and cook on medium heat. Add in the noodles, broth, salt, pepper, oregano, and cumin. Add the chili flakes,

Serrano chilies. Cook for 13 ½ minutes and simmer until the noodles become tender. Garnish with cilantro, sour soy cream, or avocado.

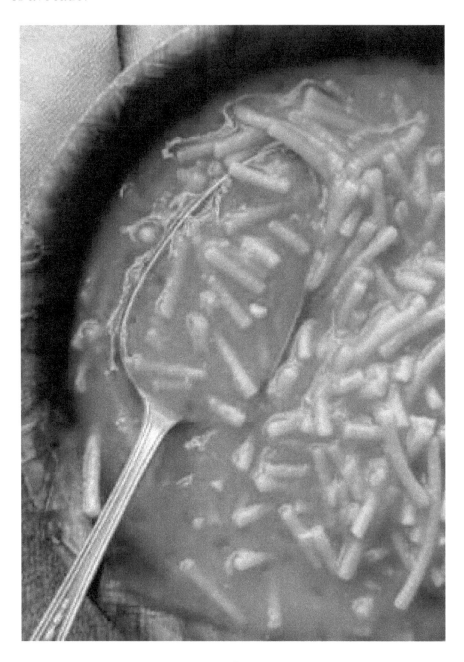

Split Pea Celery and Leek Soup

Ingredients

16- oz package

1 lb dried green split peas, rinsed

1 large leek light green and a white portion only, chopped and thoroughly cleaned

3 celery ribs diced

2 large carrots diced

4 garlic clove minced

1/4 cup chopped fresh parsley

6 cups vegetable broth

1/2 t ground black pepper

1 tsp sea salt or to taste

1 bay leaf

Directions:

Pour all of the ingredients into a slow cooker and combine thoroughly. Cover a cook on low heat for 7 and a half hours or high 3 and a half hours. Take out the bay leaf.

Red Potato and Baby Spinach Soup

Ingredients

5 cups low sodium vegetable stock

3 large red potatoes peeled and chopped

1 cup onion chopped

2 stalks celery chopped

4 cloves garlic crushed

1 cup heavy cream

1 tsp. dried tarragon

2 cups baby spinach 6-8 Tbsp. sliced almonds, sea salt, and ground black pepper to taste

Directions:

Combine stock, sweet potatoes, onion, celery, and garlic to a 4-quart slow cooker. Cook on low heat for 8 hours or until potatoes become soft. Add almond milk, tarragon, salt, and pepper. Blend this mixture for 1-2 minutes with an immersion blender until the soup is smooth. Add baby spinach & cover. Let it rest for 20 minutes or until spinach becomes soft. Garnish with almonds and season with sea salt and pepper.

Garnish with lemon Slow Cooked Lima Bean Soup

Ingredients

1 Tbsp extra virgin olive oil

6 cloves garlic, minced

1 medium red onion, diced

1/2 lb carrots, sliced thinly into rounds

4 stalks celery (1/2 bunch), sliced

1 lb dry lima beans, stones removed, rinsed, and drained

1 whole bay leaf

1 tsp dried rosemary

1/2 tsp dried thyme

1/2 tsp Spanish paprika Freshly cracked pepper (15-20 cranks of a pepper mill)

1 1/2 tsp salt or more to taste

Directions:

Put the olive oil, garlic, onion, celery, and carrots into the slow cooker. Add the beans, bay leaf, rosemary, thyme, paprika, and some freshly cracked pepper to the slow cooker. Add 6 cups of water to the slow cooker and combine the ingredients. Cover and cook for 8 hours on low or on high for 4 1/2 hours. Once it's cooked, stir the soup and mash the beans. Season with more sea salt, if necessary.

Carrot and Cardamom Soup

Ingredients

1 large red onion, finely chopped

4 fat garlic cloves, crushed

1 large carrot, finely chopped thumb-sized piece of ginger, peeled and finely chopped

2 tbsp olive oil Pinch of turmeric Seeds from 10 cardamom pods

1 tsp cumin, seeds, or ground

¼ pound soy beans

1 ¾ cup coconut milk zest and juice

1 lemon pinch of chili flakes handful of parsley, chopped

Directions:

Heat some oil in a pan and cook the onions, garlic, carrot, and ginger until softened. Add in the turmeric, cardamom, and cumin. Cook for a few mins more until the spices become aromatic. Add the soy beans, coconut milk, 1 cup of water. Boil and reduce to a simmer for 15 mins until the soy beans become soft. A process with a hand blender, pulse the soup until it's chunky. Garnish with lemon zest and juice. Season with salt, chili, and herbs. Divide among bowls and sprinkle with more lemon zest.

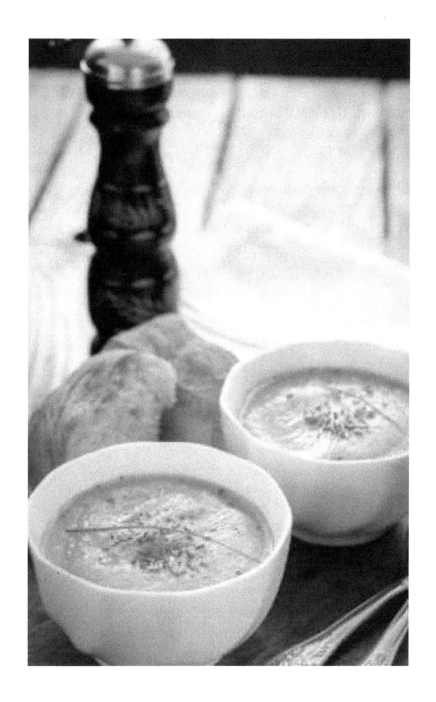

Borlotti Bean Soup

Ingredients

1 pound borlotti beans, sorted and rinsed

2 quarts veggie stock

1 medium red onion, diced

5 cloves of garlic, peeled and smashed

2 tsp. sea salt

1/4 tsp white pepper

2 medium sweet potatoes, diced

1 pound frozen, sliced parsnips

3/4 cup chopped sun-dried tomatoes*

1-2 tsp dried dill

3-4 tbsp fresh, minced parsley

Directions:

Place the beans, stock, onion, garlic, sea salt, and pepper in a pot. Cook them over low-medium heat. Simmer for 3-4 hours, or longer, add water as needed. As the beans become soft, add the sweet potato and simmer until the potatoes become tender. Add the carrots, tomatoes, and dill. Cook the parsnips until heated thoroughly. Add the parsley, season with additional salt and white pepper.

Lentil Soup

Ingredients

1/2 pound lentils, sorted and rinsed

½ pound fava beans sorted and rinsed

2 quarts veggie broth

1 medium red onion, diced

6 cloves of garlic, peeled and smashed

2 tsp. sea salt

1/4 tsp white pepper

2 medium potatoes, diced

1 pound frozen, sliced carrots

3/4 cup chopped sun-dried tomatoes*

1-2 tsp dried dill

3-4 tbsp fresh, minced parsley

Directions:

Place the beans, broth, red onion, garlic, sea salt, and pepper in a pot. Cook them over low-medium heat. Simmer for 3-4 hours, or longer, add water as needed. As the beans become soft, add the potato and simmer until the potatoes become tender. Add the carrots, tomatoes, and dill. Cook the carrots until heated thoroughly. Add the parsley, season with additional salt and white pepper.

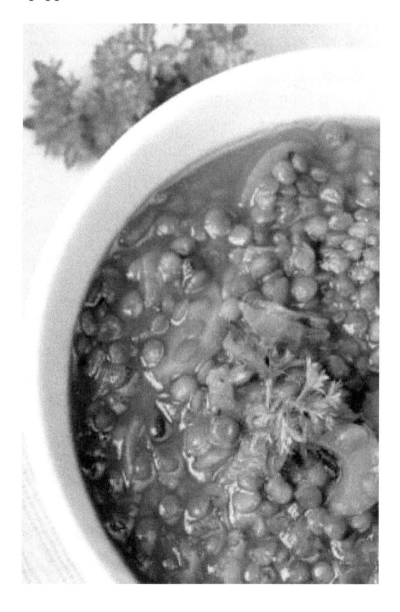

Triple Bean Soup

Ingredients

1/2 pound borlotti beans, sorted and rinsed

¼ pound great northern beans, sorted and rinsed

¼ pound kidney beans sorted and rinsed

2 quarts veggie broth

1 medium onion, diced

5 cloves of garlic, peeled and smashed

2 tsp. sea salt

1/4 tsp rainbow peppercorns

2 medium potatoes, diced

1 pound frozen, sliced carrots

3/4 cup chopped sun-dried tomatoes*

1-2 tsp dried dill

3-4 tbsp fresh, minced parsley

Directions:

Place the beans, stock, onion, garlic, sea salt, and pepper in a pot. Cook them over low-medium heat. Simmer for 3-4 hours, or longer, add water as needed. As the beans become soft, add the potato and simmer until the potatoes become tender. Add the carrots, tomatoes, and dill. Cook the carrots until heated thoroughly. Add the parsley, season with additional salt and peppercorns.

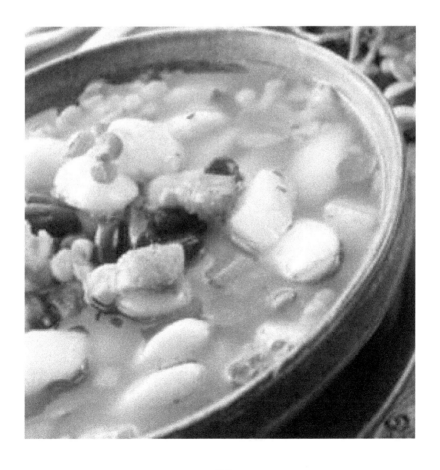

Parsnips and Summer Squash Soup

Ingredients

1 medium summer squash (1 lb of peeled and cubed butternut squash)

1/2 medium red onion, diced

½ medium yellow onion, diced

2/3 lb parsnips, peeled and cut into chunks

1 carrot, peeled and sliced

3 cups vegetable broth

1 bay leaf

1 tsp sea salt

1 tsp white pepper

1/4 tsp dried ground sage

½ can almond milk

Directions:

Combine the squash, red and yellow onion, parsnips, apple, broth, and bay leaf in a slow cooker. Cover and cook on low for about 6 hours or until veggies are soft. Take out the bay leaf and discard. Transfer these ingredients to a blender and blend until smooth Pour it back to the slow cooker, season with salt, pepper & sage. Pour the almond milk. Add more salt and pepper to taste.

Butternut Squash and Apple Soup

Ingredients

1 medium butternut squash (1 lb of peeled and cubed butternut squash)

1 medium red onion, diced

2/3 lb parsnips, peeled and cut into chunks

1 Washington apple, peeled and sliced

3 cups vegetable stock

1 bay leaf

1 tsp sea salt

1 tsp white pepper

1/4 tsp dried ground sage

½ can use coconut milk

Directions:

Combine the squash, red onion, carrots, apple, stock, and bay leaf in a slow cooker. Cover and cook on low for about 6 hours or until veggies are soft. Take out the bay leaf and discard. Transfer these ingredients to a blender and blend until smooth Pour it back to the slow cooker, season with sea salt, pepper & sage. Pour the coconut milk.

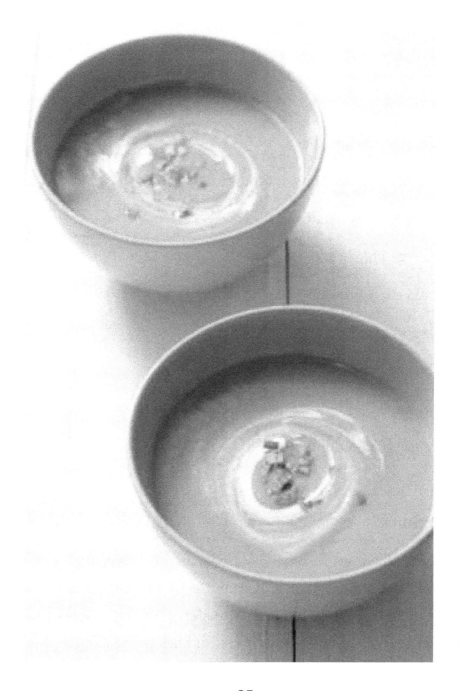

Summer Squash and Apple Soup

Ingredients

1 medium summer squash (1 lb of peeled and cubed butternut squash)

1 medium red onion, diced

2/3 lb carrots, peeled and cut into chunks

1 Fuji apple, peeled and sliced

3 cups vegetable broth

1 tsp. red curry powder

1 tsp sea salt

1 tsp black pepper

1/4 tsp cumin

½ can use coconut milk

Directions:

Combine the squash, onion, carrots, apple, broth, and curry powder in a slow cooker. Cover and cook on low for about 6 hours or until veggies are soft. Transfer these ingredients to a blender and blend until smooth Pour it back to the slow cooker, season with salt, pepper & cumin. Pour the coconut milk. Add more salt and pepper to taste.

Chinese Butternut Squash Soup

Ingredients

1 medium butternut squash (1 lb of peeled and cubed butternut squash)

1 medium red onion, diced

2/3 lb carrots, peeled and cut into chunks

1 pear, peeled and sliced

3 cups vegetable broth

2 tbsp. sesame seed oil

1 tsp sea salt

1 tsp Sichuan peppercorns

1/4 tsp dried ground sage

½ can almond milk

Directions:

Combine the squash, onion, carrots, pear & broth in a slow cooker. Cover and cook on low for about 6 hours or until veggies are soft. Take out the bay leaf and discard. Transfer these ingredients to a blender and blend until smooth Pour it back to the slow cooker, season with salt, pepper, sesame oil & Sichuan peppercorns. Pour the almond milk. Add more salt and pepper to taste.

Pinto Beans and Olives Tortilla Soup

Ingredients:

1 teaspoon extra-virgin olive oil

1/2 cup chopped red onions

6 cloves garlic, minced

1 cup vegetable broth

1 cup vegetable stock

1 cup salsa

1 14-ounce can pinto beans

5 pcs. black olives

5 pcs. capers

1 green bell pepper, chopped

1/2 teaspoon salt

1 avocado, chopped

1/2 cup loosely-packed cilantro

Optional: 1/2 cup crumbled corn tortilla chips Add olive oil to a pan and heat it to medium.

Directions:

Add onions and garlic to the saucepan and sauté until softened. Add the stock, salsa, bell peppers, capers, olives beans, and salt. Bring to a boil over high heat. Reduce to low and simmer for 5 minutes. Garnish with half of the avocado, cilantro, and tortilla chips.

Butterbean Taco Soup

Ingredients:

1 teaspoon extra-virgin olive oil

1/2 cup chopped red onions

8 cloves garlic, minced

1 lime, peeled

1 cup vegetable broth

1 cup vegetable stock

1 cup salsa

1 14-ounce can of butterbeans

1 green bell pepper, chopped

1/2 teaspoon salt

1 avocado, chopped

1/2 cup loosely-packed cilantro

Directions:

Add red onions and garlic to the saucepan and sauté until softened. Add the stock, salsa, bell peppers, beans, lime, and salt. Bring to a boil over high heat. Reduce to low and simmer for 5 minutes. Garnish with half of the avocado, cilantro, and tortilla chips. Remove the lime.

Jalapeno and Soybean Taco Soup

Ingredients:

1 teaspoon olive oil

1/2 cup chopped red onions

10 cloves garlic, minced

1 cup vegetable broth

1 cup vegetable stock

1 cup salsa

1 14-ounce can eat soy beans

1 green bell pepper, chopped

1 Anaheim pepper, coarsely chopped

2 jalapeno peppers, coarsely chipped

1/2 teaspoon salt

1 avocado, chopped

1/2 cup loosely-packed cilantro

Directions:

Optional: 1/2 cup crumbled corn tortilla chips Add olive oil to a pan and heat it to medium. Add red onions and garlic to the saucepan and sauté until softened. Add the stock, salsa, bell peppers, Anaheim peppers, jalapeno, beans, and salt. Bring to a boil over high heat. Reduce to low and simmer for 5 minutes. Garnish with half of the avocado, cilantro, and tortilla chips.

Navy Bean and Jalapeno Pepper Soup

Ingredients:

1 teaspoon olive oil

1/2 cup chopped red onions

4 cloves garlic, minced

1 cup vegetable broth

1 cup vegetable stock

1 cup salsa

1 14-ounce can navy beans

1 green bell pepper, chopped

1 jalapeno pepper, coarsely chopped

1/2 teaspoon sea salt

1 avocado, chopped

1/2 cup loosely-packed cilantro

Directions:

Optional: 1/2 cup crumbled corn tortilla chips Add olive oil to a pan and heat it to medium. Add red onions and garlic to the saucepan and sauté until softened. Add the stock, salsa, bell peppers, jalapeno, beans, and sea salt. Bring to a boil over high heat. Reduce to low and simmer for 5 minutes. Garnish with half of the avocado, cilantro, and tortilla chips.

Pigeon Peas Soup

(Prep time: 10 min| Cooking Time: 20 min| Serve: 2)

Ingredients

½ tablespoon butter

1 tablespoon fresh ginger, peeled and finely chopped

1 tablespoon garlic, minced

½ large onion, finely chopped

1 parsnip, peeled and finely diced

½ cup broccoli

½ teaspoon salt

½ cup unsweetened soy milk

2 cups water

½ cup dried pigeon peas, picked over and rinsed

1 tablespoon finely chopped parsley leaves for garnish

Instructions

In an Instant Pot, press Sauté and melt the butter. Add the onion, ginger, garlic, parsnip, and broccoli. Sauté until the vegetables are tender, about 5 minutes.

48

Add the water, soy milk, pigeon peas and season with salt and lock lid in place, and turn the valve to Sealing. Press Manual or Pressure Cooker; cook at High Pressure 15 minutes. When cooking is complete, use Natural-release for 10 minutes, then release remaining pressure. Let the soup cool slightly, then puree the soup in a blender until smooth.

Ladle soup into 2 bowls and garnish with chopped parsley.

Nutrition Facts

Calories 159, Total Fat 4.3g, Saturated Fat 2g, Cholesterol 8mg, Sodium 649mg, Total Carbohydrate

25.3g, Dietary Fiber 5.9g, Total Sugars 5.7g, Protein 6.1g

Chia Seeds Tomato Soup

(Prep time: 05 min| Cooking Time: 10 min| Serve: 2)

Ingredients

4 tomatoes, chopped

½ cup chia seeds

½ tablespoon butter

½ teaspoon garlic powder

½ small onion, roughly chopped

½ small zucchini, roughly chopped

1 1/2 cups vegetable broth

Salt and black pepper to taste

Instructions

Put Instant Pot on Sauté mode High and when hot, add the butter. Now add garlic powder and onion to fry, sauté well till onions soften.

Now add zucchini and chia seeds and fry for a minute.

Add in the tomatoes and mix well. Fry for 3 mines.

Now add in broth, salt, and pepper. Mix them well.

Lock lid in place and turn the valve to Sealing. Do Manual Low Pressure for 2 min. 7. When cooking is complete, use Natural-release for 10 minutes, then release remaining pressure. 8. Blend the chia seeds tomato mixture into a smooth puree.

If desired, adjust the consistency of the soup. Serve hot.

Nutrition Facts

Calories116, Total Fat 5.8g, Saturated Fat 2.2g, Cholesterol 8mg, Sodium 303mg, Total Carbohydrate 13.5g, Dietary Fiber 5.4g, Total Sugars 6.4g, Protein 4.7g

Zucchini Soup

(Prep time: 05 min| Cooking Time: 10 min| Serve: 2)

Ingredients

¼ medium onion diced

1 teaspoon coconut oil

1 teaspoon garlic powder

2 zucchini, peeled and cut into 4-inch chunks

½ sweet potato

½ cup almond milk

2 cups vegetable broth

1 teaspoon salt

½ teaspoon pepper

Instructions

Select the Sauté function to heat the Instant Pot. When the pot displays −Hot‖, add the coconut oil, onion, and garlic powder. Sauté until the onion softens. Press Cancel to turn off the sauté function.

Add the zucchini, sweet potato, almond milk, broth, salt, and pepper. Stir well. Lock lid in place and turn the valve to Sealing. Press the Pressure Cooker button and set the time to 10 minutes.

Once cooking is complete, turn the valve to the Venting position to release the pressure. When all the pressure is released, carefully remove the lid.

Stir the soup. Blend with an immersion blender or in batches in a stand blender until smooth.

Serve hot.

Nutrition Facts

Calories277, Total Fat 16.5g, Saturated Fat 13.2g, Cholesterol 0mg, Sodium 1986mg, Total Carbohydrate 26g, Dietary Fiber 7.2g, Total Sugars 12.3g, Protein 12.1g

Anise Seed and Cabbage Soup

(Prep time: 10 min| Cooking Time: 15 min| Serve: 2)

Ingredients

½ tablespoon olive oil

½ onion

½ teaspoon garlic minced

½ tablespoon anise seed

½ pound cabbage

½ cup almond milk

2 cups vegetable broth

½ teaspoon salt and black pepper for serving

Instructions

Select the Sauté function to heat the Instant Pot. When the pot displays —Hot‖, add the olive oil, onion, and garlic. Sauté until the onion softens.

Add the cabbage, anise seed, almond milk, broth, salt, and pepper. Stir well. Lock lid in place and turn the valve to Sealing. Press the Pressure Cooker button and set the time to10 minutes.

Once cooking is complete, turn the valve to the Venting position to release the pressure. When all the pressure is released, carefully remove the lid.

Use a standing blender or an immersion blender to puree the soup to a smooth, creamy consistency.

Serve.

Nutrition Facts

Calories253, Total Fat 19.6g, Saturated Fat 13.6g, Cholesterol 0mg, Sodium 1376mg, Total Carbohydrate 14.5g, Dietary Fiber 5g, Total Sugars 7.5g, Protein 8.3g

Bok Choy Soup

(Prep time: 05 min| Cooking Time: 10 min| Serve: 2)

Ingredients

2 cups of bok choy, diced

1 celery

1 bell pepper

1 potato, peeled and diced

1.5 cups of vegetable stock

½ cup of soy milk

Salt and pepper to taste

Instructions

Add diced bok choy, celery, potato, vegetable stock, and soy milk and bell pepper into Instant Pot.

Add salt and pepper to the mixture.

Turn the Instant Pot to the −Soup‖ function and let it cook. Alternatively, put everything in a pot and bring to boil and simmer until the celeriac and potato are soft.

When cool, puree it with an immersion blender like this one or put it in a High-speed blender.

Enjoy!

Nutrition Facts

Calories 131, Total Fat 1.6g, Saturated Fat 0.2g, Cholesterol 0mg, Sodium 131mg, Total Carbohydrate

26g, Dietary Fiber 3.6g, Total Sugars 7.5g, Protein 5.8g

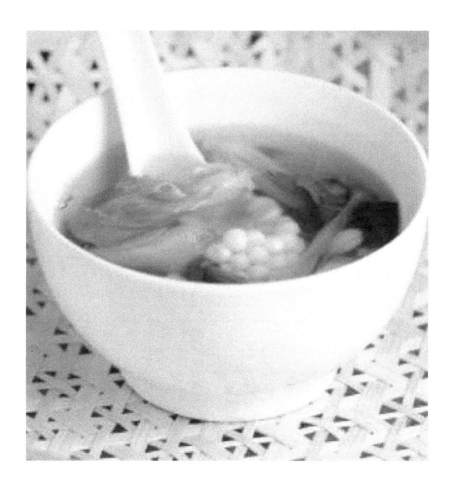

Spicy Peanut Soup with Potato and Spinach

(Prep time: 05 min| Cooking Time: 10 min| Serve: 2)

Ingredients

½ tablespoons butter

½ onion, diced

1 bell pepper, minced

1 teaspoon garlic, minced

1 potato, peeled and cubed

1 tomato

½ cup coconut milk

2 cups vegetable broth

1 teaspoon salt

½ teaspoon turmeric

1/8 cup chopped peanuts

1 teaspoon peanut butter

1 cup spinach, chopped

Instructions

Select the Sauté function to heat the instant Pot inner pot. When the pot displays —Hot‖, add butter, onion, and garlic. Sauté until the onion softens. Add the bell pepper, potato, tomatoes, coconut milk, broth, turmeric, peanuts, salt, and pepper. Stir them well. Lock lid in place and turn the valve to Sealing. Press the Pressure Cooker button and set the time to10 minutes.

Once cooking is complete, turn the valve to the Venting position to release the pressure. When all the pressure is released, carefully remove the lid.

Add spinach and peanut butter into the mixer. Use a standing blender or an immersion blender to puree the soup to a smooth, creamy consistency.

Serve.

Nutrition Facts

Calories 386, Total Fat 24.9g, Saturated Fat 15.9g, Cholesterol 8mg, Sodium 1992mg, Total Carbohydrate 32.6g, Dietary Fiber 7.1g, Total Sugars 9.6g, Protein 12.8g

Parsnip Ginger Soup with Tofu and Kale

(Prep time: 10 min| Cooking Time: 20 min| Serve: 2)

Ingredients

½ tablespoon butter

1 small onion, diced

1 teaspoon ginger powder

1 teaspoon garlic powder

½ pound parsnip, cut into small coins

½ teaspoon cumin

½ teaspoon ground coriander

¼ teaspoon ground turmeric

1 1/2 cups of vegetable broth

½ cup of soy milk

½ teaspoon honey

½ fresh lime

1 cup tofu, diced into cubes

1 handful of fresh kale

Instructions

Set the Instant Pot to Sauté and add butter, add tofu cook it for 5 min. Keep aside.

After add onions. Cook for 5-10 minutes until the onion begins to soften.

Add the garlic and ginger powder to the pot and stir until fragrant.

Combine the parsnip, cumin, coriander powder, and turmeric powder in the Instant Pot. Stir well.

Pour in the broth and lock the lid. Turn the vent to seal, press Cancel, and manually cook on High Pressure for 5 minutes.

After 5 minutes, do a manual release.

Add the soy milk and honey if using to the Instant Pot. Allow the mixture to cool slightly, and then use an immersion blender or other mixer to puree until smooth. Season with salt, pepper, and a squeeze of lime.

Stir the fresh kale into the still, slightly warm soup. The kale should wilt on its own, but you can also warm it up together for the right temperature. Add the tofu, and enjoy!

Nutrition Facts

Calories 303, Total Fat 10.5g, Saturated Fat 3.3g, Cholesterol 8mg, Sodium

478mg, Total Carbohydrate 38.9g, Dietary Fiber 9.2g, Total Sugars 12.6g, Protein 18.1g

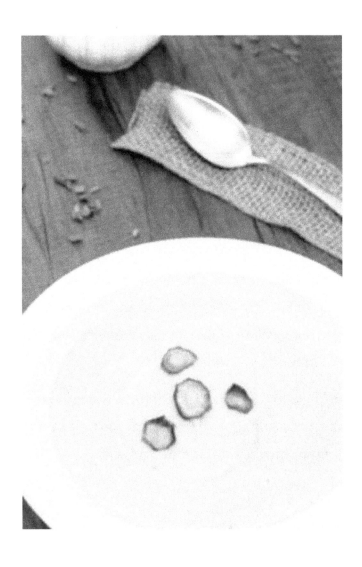

Mushroom Soup

(Prep time: 10 min| Cooking Time: 25 min| Serve: 2)

Ingredients

1 teaspoon avocado oil

½ medium onion, chopped

½ large leek stalk, chopped

½ large zucchini peeled & chopped

1 teaspoon garlic powder

8 ounces mushrooms sliced

½ teaspoon dried rosemary

¼ teaspoon ground pepper

1 1/2 cups vegetable broth

¼ teaspoon salt

½ cup almond milk

Instructions

Set the Instant Pot to Sauté mode. Heat the avocado oil, then add the onion, leek, and zucchini. Sauté the vegetables, occasionally stirring, until starting to soften, 3 to 4 minutes.

Add the garlic powder, mushrooms, rosemary, and pepper. Cook until the mushrooms are starting to release their liquid, 2 to 3 minutes. Stir in the broth and salt.

Put the lid on the Instant Pot, close the steam vent, and set it to High Pressure using the Manual setting. Decrease the time to 10 minutes. It will take the Instant Pot about 10 minutes to reach pressure.

Once the time is up, carefully release the steam using the Quick-release valve.

Transfer half of the soup to the blender, add the almond milk, hold on the top and blend until almost smooth, stop the blender, and occasionally open the lid to release the steam. Transfer the pureed soup to a pot or bowl.

Nutrition Facts

Calories228, Total Fat 15.9g, Saturated Fat 13g, Cholesterol 0mg, Sodium 702mg, Total Carbohydrate

17.5g, Dietary Fiber 4.8g, Total Sugars 8.1g, Protein 9.3g

Seitan Stew with Barley

(Prep time: 10 min| Cooking Time: 20 min| Serve: 2)

Ingredients

1 teaspoon coconut oil

½ onion chopped

1 parsnip cut into thin half-circles

1 leek stalks diced

1 teaspoon garlic minced

1 teaspoon dried basil

½ teaspoons dried parsley

1 1/2 tablespoons tomato paste

2 cups vegetable broth

1 cup seitan

1 cup dry barley

½ teaspoon salt

½ teaspoon ground pepper

Instructions

Set the Instant Pot to Sauté mode. Heat the coconut oil, then add the onion, parsnips, and leek. Sauté the vegetables, occasionally stirring, until starting to soften, 3 to 4 minutes.

Add the garlic, basil, parsley, and tomato paste. Cook, constantly stirring, for 1 minute. Pour in the vegetable broth and stir to combine. Add the seitan, barley, and salt and pepper to the Instant Pot.

Put the lid on the Instant Pot, close the steam vent, and set it to High Pressure using the Manual setting. Set the time to 20 minutes. Once the time is expired, use Natural-release for 10 minutes, then quickly release.

Serve soup with salt and pepper to taste.

Nutrition Facts

Calories 376, Total Fat 5.8g, Saturated Fat 2.9g, Cholesterol 0mg, Sodium 1600mg, Total Carbohydrate 57.9g, Dietary Fiber 13.7g, Total Sugars 8.2g, Protein 23.5g

Cottage Cheese Soup

(Prep time: 10 min| Cooking Time: 35 min| Serve: 2)

Ingredients

1 stalks leek, diced

1 tablespoon bell pepper, diced

¼ cup Swiss chard, sliced into strips

1/8 cup fresh kale

1 eggplant

½ tablespoon avocado oil

1/8 cup button mushrooms, diced

1 small onion, diced

½ cup cottage cheese

2 cups vegetable broth

1 bay leaf

½ teaspoon salt

¼ teaspoon garlic, minced

1/8 teaspoon paprika

Instructions

Place leek, bell pepper, Swiss chard, eggplant, and kale into a medium bowl, set aside in a separate medium bowl. Press the Sauté button and add the avocado oil to Instant Pot. Once the oil is hot, add mushrooms and onion. Sauté for 4–6 minutes until onion is translucent and fragrant. Add leek, bell pepper, Swiss chard, and kale to Instant Pot. Cook for additional 4 minutes. Press the Cancel button.

Add diced cottage cheese, broth, bay leaf, and seasonings to Instant Pot. Click lid closed. Press the Soup button and set the time for 20 minutes.

When the timer beeps, allow a 10-minute natural release and quickly release the remaining pressure. Add eggplant on Keep Warm mode and cook for additional 10 minutes or until tender. Serve warm.

Nutrition Facts

Calories 212, Total Fat 3.6g, Saturated Fat 1.2g, Cholesterol 5mg, Sodium 1603mg, Total Carbohydrate

30.7g, Dietary Fiber 11.9g, Total Sugars 12.7g, Protein 17g

Cauliflower Soup

(Prep time: 10 min| Cooking Time: 5 min| Serve: 2)

Ingredients

5 cups vegetable broth or water

1 medium onion chopped

1 - 2 stalks leek thinly sliced

2 cloves garlic crushed

1 lb. cauliflower cut in big chunks

1 teaspoon salt

1/2 teaspoon pepper

1 teaspoon fresh basil

1/4 cup almond flour

2/3 cup water

1 cup grated goat cheese

1/2 cup milk

Salt and pepper to taste

Instructions

Add the first 8 ingredients (including basil) to the Instant Pot and lock lid. Make sure the valve is set to Sealing and press Pressure Cooker (or Manual). Set the time with the + /- button for 5 minutes.

While cooking, stir in flour and water until smooth. When the IP beeps, flip the valve from Sealing to Venting, and when the pin drops, press Cancel and remove the lid.

Press the Sauté button and cook again, stirring frequently. Whisk the flour-water mixture and add about half of it to the soup.

Use a hand blender to puree the soup. Or use a blender or food processor and put it back in the pan.

Press Cancel and add the cheese. Stir until melted. Do not cook after the cheese has gone in. Add the milk, salt, and pepper to your taste. Serve with a pinch of grated cheese.

Nutrition Facts

Calories 202, Total Fat 8.4g, Saturated Fat 4.4g, Cholesterol 20mg, Sodium 1345mg, Total Carbohydrate 23.2g, Dietary Fiber 7.8g, Total Sugars 11.3g, Protein 12.6g

Pumpkin Soup

(Prep time: 10 min| Cooking Time: 20 min| Serve: 2)

Ingredients

1 lb pumpkin peeled and seeded 1/2-1- inch cubes

1 cup vegetable broth or water

1 teaspoon dried rosemary

1/4 teaspoon grated cinnamon

1/2 teaspoon salt

1 cup coconut milk

2 tablespoons butter

1 tablespoon almond flour

Instructions

Mix the pumpkin cubes, broth, rosemary, cinnamon, and salt in an Instant Pot. Lock the lid onto the pot.

Press Soup/Broth, Pressure Cooker, or Manual on High Pressure for 5 minutes with the Keep Warm setting off. The valve must be closed. Use the Quick-release mode to return the pot pressure to normal. Unlock the lid and open the pot. Add coconut milk.

Use an immersion blender to puree the soup right in the pot. Or work in halves to puree the soup in a covered blender. If necessary, pour all the soup back into the pan.

Press the Sauté button and set it for Low, 250°F. Set the timer for 5 minutes.

Bring the soup to a simmer, stirring often. In the meantime, place the butter in a small bowl or measuring container and place it in the microwave in 5-second increments. Use a fork to mix the flour and make a thin paste.

When the soup is boiling, Whisk the butter mixture into the pan. Continue whisking until the soup is a bit thick, about 1 minute. Turn off the Sauté function and allow it to cool for a few minutes before serving.

Nutrition Facts

Calories 415, Total Fat 41g, Saturated Fat 32.9g, Cholesterol 31mg, Sodium 1064mg, Total Carbohydrate 11.5g, Dietary Fiber 3.3g, Total Sugars 5.2g, Protein 5.9g

Vegetarian Spinach Soup

(Prep time: 15 min| Cooking Time: 20 min| Serve: 2)

Ingredients

½ tablespoon coconut oil

¼ onion, finely chopped

½ stalk leek, finely chopped

1 teaspoon garlic powder

1 teaspoon basil, freshly chopped

¼ teaspoon red pepper flakes (optional)

Salt

Freshly ground black pepper

2 cups vegetable broth

Enough water

1 (15.5oz.) can chickpea, drained and rinsed

Juice of 1 lemon

1 large bunch of Spinach, removed from stems and torn into medium pieces

Instructions

In an Instant Pot, press the Sauté button and set it for Medium, heat oil. Add onion, leek, and cook until slightly soft, 6 minutes. Add garlic powder, basil, and red pepper flakes and cook until fragrant, 1 minute more. Season with salt and pepper.

Add broth, water, lemon juice, chickpea, and Spinach. Press Soup/Broth, Pressure Cooker, or Manual on High Pressure for 10 minutes with the Keep Warm setting off. The valve must be closed.

Use the Quick-release method to return the pot pressure to normal. Unlock the lid and open the pot.

Use an immersion blender to puree the soup right in the pot.

Press the Sauté button and set it for Low, 250°F. Set the timer for 5 minutes.

Bring the soup to a simmer, stirring often.

Serve.

Nutritions:

50.7g, Dietary Fiber 15.2g, Total Sugars 9.8g, Protein 20.1g

Green Soup

(Prep time: 10 min| Cooking Time: 35 min| Serve: 2)

Ingredients

4 cups vegetable broth

1 small onion, cut into 3/4- inch pieces

1/3 cup rice

1 tablespoon vegetable oil

1 teaspoon garlic powder

Salt

1/4 cup Greek yogurt

1 tsp minced fresh mint

1/4 tsp finely grated lime zest plus 1/2 tsp juice

6 oz. collard greens stemmed and chopped

4 oz spinach, stemmed and chopped

1 cup beet greens

Instructions

Add broth, onion, rice, oil, garlic powder, and 1/2 teaspoon salt to a blender. Lock lid in place, the particular Soup program 2 (for creamy soups).

In the meantime, combine Greek yogurt, mint, lime zest, and juice, and remaining 1/4 teaspoon salt in a bowl; refrigerate until ready to serve.

Pause program 12 minutes before it has been completed. Carefully remove the lid and stir in collard greens and spinach until wholly submerged.

Return lid and resume program. Pause the program 1 minute before it has been completed. Stir in beet greens.

Return lid and resume program. Once the program has completed, adjust soup consistency with extra broth as needed and season with salt and pepper to taste. Drizzle individual portions with yogurt sauce before serving.

Nutrition Facts

Calories 306, Total Fat 9.7g, Saturated Fat 1.8g, Cholesterol 1mg 0%, Sodium 225mg, Total Carbohydrate 48.7g, Dietary Fiber 12.6g, Total Sugars 3.4g, Protein 13.6g

Zoodles Greek Salad

Prep Time 10 mins Cook Time 0 mins Servings: 4 -6

Ingredients

Juice of a lemon (about 1/4 cup)

1 Tablespoon balsamic vinegar

1 Tablespoon olive oil

1 teaspoon minced fresh oregano kosher salt & pepper

2 medium zucchini (peeled if desired)

1 cup grape or cherry tomatoes, halved

1/2 cup pitted kalamata olives, halved

2 oz. crumbled feta cheese (about 1/2 cup)

Instructions

In a small bowl, whisk together the lemon juice, balsamic vinegar, olive oil, oregano, and salt and pepper, to taste, and set the dressing aside.

Using, a vegetable spiral cutter, cut the zucchini into zucchini noodles.

In a large bowl, gently toss together the zucchini noodles, tomatoes, olives, feta and the dressing until combined and evenly coated.

Nutrition Info

Calories: 121kcal Carbohydrates: 6g Protein: 3g

Fat: 9g

Saturated Fat: 3g Cholesterol: 12mg Sodium: 433mg Potassium: 336mg Fiber: 2g

Sugar: 4g

Antipasto Cauliflower Salad

Servings: (8) 1/2 cup

Ingredients

2 cups of raw cauliflower, chopped

1/2 cup radicchio, chopped

1/2 cup artichoke hearts, chopped

1/3 cup fresh basil, chopped

1/2 cup freshly grated parmesan

3 Tbsp sundried tomatoes, chopped

3 Tbsp kalamata olives, chopped

1 clove garlic, minced

3 Tbsp balsamic vinegar

3 Tbsp extra virgin olive oil salt and pepper to taste

Instructions

First, cook your finely chopped cauliflower in the microwave for five minutes. Don't add any liquid or seasoning to it, just spread it on a microwave safe dish and zap it. Let the cauliflower cool while you prep the other ingredients.

Combine the radicchio, artichoke hearts, basil, parmesan, sundried tomatoes, olives, and garlic in a medium bowl.

In a smaller bowl, whisk together the olive oil and vinegar, then pour it over the salad. Toss to combine, and season with salt and pepper to taste. Can be served room temperature or chilled.

Nutrition Info

Calories: 102 Fat: 8g

Carbohydrates: 4g net Protein: 3g

Charred Veggie and Fried Goat Cheese Salad

Servings 2

Ingredients

2 tablespoons poppy seeds

2 tablespoons sesame seeds 1 teaspoon onion flakes

1 teaspoon garlic flakes

4 ounces goat cheese, cut into

4 ½ in thick medallions

1 medium red bell pepper, seeds removed & cut into 8 pieces

½ cup baby portobello mushrooms, sliced

4 cups arugula, divided between two bowls

1 tablespoon avocado oil

Instructions

Combine the poppy and sesame seeds, onion, and garlic flakes in a small dish.

Coat each piece of goat cheese on both sides. Plate and place in the refrigerator until you are ready to fry the cheese. Prepare a skillet with nonstick spray and heat to medium. Char the peppers and mushrooms on both sides, just until the pieces begin to darken and the pepper softens. Add to the bowls of arugula.

Place the cold goat cheese in the skillet and fry on each side for about 30 seconds. This melts quickly so be gentle as you flip each piece!

Add the cheese to the salad and drizzle with avocado oil. Serve warm!

Nutrition Info

350 Calories

27.61 g Fat

7.08 g Net Carbs

16.09 g Protein.

Simple Greek Salad

This Simple Greek Salad comes together in under five minutes. By using a few key flavors you can whip up a restaurant quality side in no time.

Prep Time: 10 minutes Total Time: 10 minutes Servings: 6

Ingredients

1 cucumbers peeled and chopped

1 pint grape tomatoes halved

4 oz feta cheese cubed

2 tbsp fresh dill

2 tbsp extra virgin olive oil

Instructions

Combine the first four ingredients in a medium bowl. Drizzle with the olive oil. Toss lightly to combine.

Nutrition Info

Calories: 117 Carbohydrates: 6g Protein: 4g

Fat: 9g Saturated Fat: 4g Cholesterol: 17mg Sodium: 217mg Potassium: 335mg Fiber: 2g

Sugar: 4g

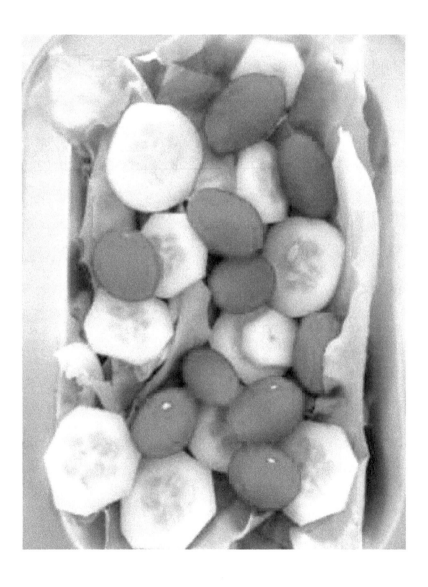

Keto Asian Noodle Salad with Peanut Sauce

This easy vegetarian Keto Asian Noodle Salad can be made in advance for picnics, parties, or as meal prep for keto lunches all week! Low carb, Atkins, Paleo, gluten free, and can easily be made vegan

Prep Time: 10 minutes Total Time: 10 minutes Servings: 4 servings

Ingredients

For the salad:

1 cup shredded red cabbage

1 cup shredded green cabbage 1/4 cup chopped scallions

1/4 cup chopped cilantro

4 cups shiritake noodles (drained and rinsed) 1/4 cup chopped peanuts

For the dressing:

2 tablespoons minced ginger 1 teaspoon minced garlic

½ cup filtered water

1 tablespoon lime juice

1 tablespoon toasted sesame oil

1 tablespoon wheat-free soy sauce

1 tablespoon fish sauce (or coconut aminos for vegan)

¼ cup sugar free peanut butter

¼ teaspoon cayenne pepper

½ teaspoon kosher salt

1 tablespoon granulated erythritol sweetener

Instructions

Combine all of the salad ingredients in a large bowl.

Combine all of the dressing ingredients in a blender or magic bullet.

Blend until smooth. Pour the dressing over the salad and toss to coat.

Serve immediately, or store in an airtight container in the refrigerator for up to 5 days. Do not freeze.

Nutrition Info

Serving Size: 1.5 cups Calories: 212

Fat: 16g Carbohydrates: 9g Fiber: 3g

Protein: 7g

Crispy Tofu and Bok Choy Salad

Servings 3 servings

Ingredients

Oven Baked Tofu

15 ounces extra firm tofu

1 tablespoon soy sauce

1 tablespoon sesame oil

1 tablespoon water

2 teaspoons minced garlic

1 tablespoon rice wine vinegar

Juice ½ lemon

Bok Choy Salad

9 ounces bok choy

1 stalk green onion

2 tablespoons chopped cilantro

3 tablespoons coconut oil

2 tablespoons soy sauce 1 tablespoon sambal olek

1 tablespoon peanut butter

Juice ½ lime

7 drops liq uid stevia

Instructions

Start by pressing the tofu. Lay the tofu in a kitchen towel and put something heavy over the top (like a cast iron skillet). It takes about 4-6 hours to dry out, and you may need to replace the kitchen towel half-way through.

Once the tofu is pressed, work on your marinade. Combine all of the ingredients for the marinade (soy sauce, sesame oil, water, garlic, vinegar, and lemon).

Chop the tofu into sq uares and place in a plastic bag along with the marinade. Let this marinate for at least 30 minutes, but preferably over night.

Pre-heat oven to 350°F. Place tofu on a baking sheet lined with parchment paper (or a silpat) and bake for 30-35 minutes.

As the tofu is cooked, get started on the bok choy salad. Chop cilantro and spring onion.

Mix all of the other ingredients together (except lime juice and bok choy) in a bowl. Then add cilantro and spring onion. Note:

You can microwave coconut oil for 10-15 seconds to allow it it to melt.

Once the tofu is almost cooked, add lime juice into the salad dressing and mix together.

Chop the bok choy into small slices, like you would cabbage. Remove the tofu from the oven and assemble your salad with tofu, bok choy, and sauce. Enjoy!

Low-Carb Snap Pea Salad

This Low-Carb Snap Pea Salad makes a perfect side dish for Spring. It is suitable for low-carb, Atkins, LC/HF, gluten-free, and Banting diets.

Prep Time 5 minutes Cook Time 10 minutes Total Time 40 minutes Servings 4

Ingredients

8 ounces cauliflower riced

1/4 cup lemon juice

1/4 cup olive oil

1 clove garlic crushed

1/2 teaspoon coarse grain dijon mustard

1 teaspoon granulated stevia/erythritol blend

1/4 teaspoon pepper

1/2 teaspoon sea salt

1/2 cup sugar snap peas ends removed and each pod cut into three pieces

1/4 cup chives

1/2 cup sliced almonds 1/4 cup red onions minced

Instructions

Pour 1 to 2 inches of water in a pot fitted with a steamer. Bring water to a simmer.

Place riced cauliflower in the steamer basket, sprinkle lightly with sea salt, cover, and place over the simmering water in the bottom of the steamer. Steam until tender, about 10-12 minutes. When cauliflower is tender, remove the top of the steamer from the simmering water and place it over a bowl, so any excess water can drain out. Allow to cool, uncovered for about 10 minutes, then cover and place the steamer and the bowl in the refrigerator. Chill for at least 1/2 hour or until cool to the touch. While cauliflower is cooling, make the dressing. Pour olive oil in a small mixing bowl. Gradually stream in the lemon juice while vigorously whisking. Whisk in the garlic, mustard, sweetener, pepper, and salt.

In a medium mixing bowl, combine chilled cauliflower, peas, chives, almonds, and red onions. Pour dressing over and stir to mix. Transfer to an airtight container and refrigerate until serving. This salad is best if it is allowed to sit for a few hours in the refrigerator so the flavors mingle.

Nutrition Info

Calories: 212

Fat (g): 20

Carbs (g): 6

Fiber (g): 2 Protein (g):

Net Carbs (g): 4

Black Bean Salad with Apricots

(Prep time: 15 min| Cooking Time: 15 min | serve: 2)

Ingredients

½ cup apricots, finely chopped

½ green bell pepper, finely chopped

¼ red onion, finely diced

½ cup black beans

½ cup finely chopped fresh rosemary

1/2 teaspoon ground cumin

Sea salt to taste

½ avocado, peeled, pitted, and chopped

2 tablespoons lime juice

2 teaspoons coconut oil

Lime juice

2 cups water

Instructions

Pour black beans and water into Instant Pot. Lock the lid into place. Select Pressure Cook or Manual, and adjust the pressure to High and the time to 10 minutes. After cooking, let the pressure release naturally for 2 minutes, then quickly release any remaining pressure.

Mix apricots, green bell pepper, and onions in a bowl; gently fold in black beans and rosemary. Season with ground cumin and sea salt. Fold in avocado and drizzle salad with lime juice and coconut oil. Let stand for 5-10 minutes before serving.

Nutrition Facts

Calories 426, Total Fat 17.7g, Saturated Fat 7.2g, Cholesterol 0mg, Sodium 133mg, Total Carbohydrate 53.6g, Dietary Fiber 18.5g, Total Sugars 7.2g, Protein 13.3g

Red Potato Salad

(Prep time: 5 min| Cooking Time: 20 min | serve: 2)

Ingredients

½ cup red potatoes or gold, cut into bite-sized pieces

1 egg

¼ cup mayonnaise

½ teaspoon Dijon mustard

¼ cup dill seed

1 small onion, thinly sliced

1 tablespoon cilantro, chopped

½ cup goat cheese, grated

1 teaspoon pepper

1 1/2 cups of water

Instructions

Pour 1 1/2 cups of water into the Instant Pot and insert the steam rack. Place cubed potatoes in a steamer basket and lower the steamer basket onto the steam rack. Add an egg on top of the potatoes.

Secure the lid, making sure the vent is closed.

Use the display panel and select the Manual or Pressure Cook function. Use the + /- keys and program the Instant Pot for 5 minutes.

When the time is up, quickly release the pressure.

Remove eggs and place in an ice bath. And the potatoes and allow to cool.

Keep the egg in an ice bath for 5 minutes, then peel and chop.

Meanwhile, in a large bowl, whisk together mayonnaise and Dijon mustard. Mix in dill seed, onion, and cilantro.

Fold in cooked potatoes, chopped eggs, goat cheese, and pepper. Season to taste.

Serve chilled garnish with extra cilantro.

Nutrition Facts

Calories 272, Total Fat 15.5g, Saturated Fat 3.3g, Cholesterol 93mg, Sodium 299mg, Total Carbohydrate 25.2g, Dietary Fiber 4.9g, Total Sugars 4.5g, Protein 8.1g

Awesome Pasta Salad

(Prep time: 30min| Cooking Time: 10 min | serve: 2)

Ingredients

½ cup fusilli pasta

½ cup cherry tomatoes halved

½ cup goat cheese, cubed

1 boiled egg

½ red bell pepper, cut into 1-inch pieces

½ cup corn, drained

½ cup mayonnaise

Salt and pepper to taste

¼ teaspoon oregano

½ teaspoon garlic powder

1 1/2 cups of water

Instructions

Put fusilli pasta in an Instant Pot. Stir in the water, oregano, garlic powder until smooth. Stir. Lock the lid onto the pot. Press

Pressure Cook on Max Pressure for 5 minutes with the Keep Warm setting off.

When the Instant Pot has finished cooking, turn it off and let its pressure return naturally for 1 minute. Then use the Quick Release method to get rid of any residual pressure in the pot.

In a large bowl, combine pasta with cherry tomatoes, goat cheese, red bell pepper, egg, corn, and mayonnaise and toss to coat.

Nutrition Facts

Calories 227, Total Fat 8g, Saturated Fat 2.9g, Cholesterol 91mg, Sodium 194mg, Total Carbohydrate

29.1g, Dietary Fiber 2.8g, Total Sugars 5.2g, Protein 9.7g

Brown Lentil Salad with dill

(Prep time: 10min| Cooking Time: 20 min | serve: 2)

Ingredients

¼ cup dry brown lentils

¼ cup diced carrots

¼ cup red onion, diced

½ teaspoon garlic powder

1 bay leaf

½ teaspoon dried basil

1 tablespoon lemon juice

½ cup diced leek

¼ cup chopped mint

¼ teaspoon salt

¼ teaspoon ground black pepper

¼ cup coconut oil

1 1/2 cups of water

Instructions

Combine lentils, carrots, onion, garlic powder, bay leaf, and basil in Instant Pot. Add water. Lock the lid onto the pot. Press Pressure Cook on Max Pressure for 5 minutes with the Keep Warm setting off.

When the Instant Pot has finished cooking, turn it off and let its pressure return naturally for 1 minute. Then use the Quick Release method to get rid of any residual pressure in the pot.

Drain lentils and vegetables and remove bay leaf. Add coconut oil, lemon juice, leeks, mint, salt, and pepper. Toss to mix and serve at room temperature.

Nutrition Facts

Calories 369, Total Fat 28g, Saturated Fat 23.8g, Cholesterol 0mg, Sodium 312mg, Total Carbohydrate 22.1g, Dietary Fiber 4.7g, Total Sugars 2.5g, Protein 7.2g

Cucumber, Mango, and Barley Salad

(Prep time: 5 min| Cooking Time: 20 min | serve: 2)

Ingredients

½ cup barley

¼ teaspoon ground cumin

½ cup water

½ mango, peeled and diced

½ cucumber, seeded and diced

½ red bell pepper, seeded and diced

½ cup broccoli

½ tablespoon chopped parsley

½ lime, juiced

Salt and ground black pepper to taste

Instructions

Put barley, water, and broccoli in Instant Pot. Lock the lid into place. Select Pressure Cook or Manual, and adjust the pressure to High and the time to 15 minutes. Make sure the vent on top is set to Sealing. After cooking, naturally, release the pressure.

Unlock and remove the lid. Drain the beans and let cool for about 5 minutes. Mix mango, cucumbers, red bell peppers, chopped parsley, lime juice, salt, and black pepper in a bowl; stir in barley mixture. Serve immediately or chill in the refrigerator before serving.

Nutrition Facts

Calories 266, Total Fat 1.7g, Saturated Fat 0.3g, Cholesterol 0mg, Sodium 19mg, Total Carbohydrate 54.8g, Dietary Fiber 11.2g, Total Sugars 15.3g, Protein 8.1g

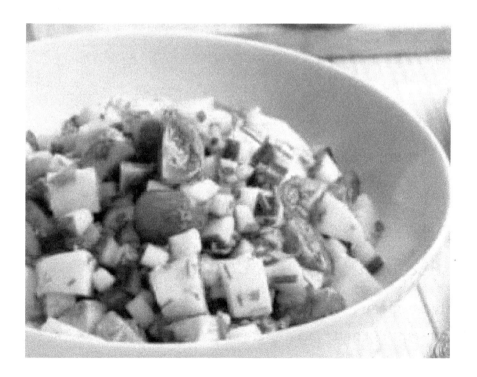

Greek Green Bean Salad with Feta and Tomatoes

(Prep time: 10 min| Cooking Time: 5 min | serve: 2)

Ingredients

1 cup fresh green beans, trimmed

2 tomatoes, chopped

1 tablespoon avocado oil

2 tablespoons vinegar

Salt and freshly ground black pepper to taste

1 onion, minced

¼ cup chopped fresh basil

1 teaspoon garlic powder

½ cup crumbled parmesan cheese

1 cup water

Instructions

Place the green beans in a steamer basket. Add 1 cup of water to the Instant Pot and place the steamer basket inside. Lock the lid into place. Select Steam and adjust the pressure to High and the time to 10 minutes. Pressure release naturally for 2 minutes, then quickly release any remaining pressure.

Combine green beans and tomatoes in a large bowl.

Stir together avocado oil, vinegar, salt, and pepper in a small bowl. Add onions, basil, and garlic powder.

Pour dressing over green beans and tomatoes and mix. Mix crumbled

parmesan cheese. Allow sitting for 20 minutes before serving.

Nutrition Facts

Calories 109, Total Fat 2.8g, Saturated Fat 1.2g, Cholesterol 5mg, Sodium 77mg, Total Carbohydrate

15.6g, Dietary Fiber 5g 18%, Total Sugars 6.7g, Protein 5.4g

Quick Edamame Salad

(Prep time: 10 min| Cooking Time: 5 min | serve: 2)

Ingredients

½ cup frozen shelled edamame

¼ cup sweet corn

¼ cup green peas

¼ cup black beans

½ red onion, minced

1 tablespoon coconut oil

½ teaspoon salt

½ teaspoon dried dill

¼ teaspoon ground black pepper

¼ teaspoon dried basil

¼ teaspoon garlic powder

1 cup water

Instructions

Place the edamame, sweet corn, black beans, peas in a steamer basket. Add 1 cup of water to the Instant Pot and place the steamer basket inside. Lock the lid into place. Select Steam and adjust the pressure to High and the time to 10 minutes. Pressure release naturally for 2 minutes, then quickly release any remaining pressure

Mix edamame, corn, peas, black beans, and red onion in a large bowl. Stir coconut oil, salt, dill, black pepper, basil, and garlic powder into an edamame mixture.

Chill in the refrigerator at least 30 minutes before serving.

Nutrition Facts

Calories 234, Total Fat 9g, Saturated Fat 6.3g, Cholesterol 0mg, Sodium 588mg, Total Carbohydrate

27.5g, Dietary Fiber 7.4g, Total Sugars 4.4g, Protein 10.8g

Green Bean and Potato Salad

(Prep time: 15 min| Cooking Time:15 min | serve: 2)

Ingredients

½ cup red potatoes

1 cup fresh green beans, trimmed and snapped

¼ cup chopped fresh basil

1 small red onion, chopped

Salt and pepper to taste

¼ cup balsamic vinegar

2 tablespoons Dijon mustard

2 tablespoons fresh lemon juice

1 teaspoon garlic powder

½ tablespoon coconut oil

Instructions

Place the potatoes in an Instant Pot, and fill with about 1-inch water. Lock the lid into place. Select Steam and adjust the pressure to High and the time to 10 minutes. Pressure release naturally for 2 minutes, quickly release any remaining pressure, add green beans to the Instant Pot. Drain, calm, and cut potatoes into quarters. Transfer to a large bowl, and toss with fresh basil, red onion, salt, and pepper. Set aside. In a medium bowl, whisk together the balsamic vinegar, mustard, lemon juice, garlic powder, and coconut oil. Pour over the salad, and stir to coat. Taste and season with additional salt and pepper if needed.

Nutrition Facts

Calories 113, Total Fat 4.3g, Saturated Fat 3.1g, Cholesterol 0mg, Sodium 189mg, Total Carbohydrate 15.7g, Dietary Fiber 4g, Total Sugars 3.6g, Protein 3.2g

CPSIA information can be obtained
at www.ICGtesting.com
Printed in the USA
BVHW092217300421
606210BV00004B/890

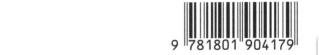